I Love My Body Series; Book 4

I Love My Skin

Natural Skincare That Actually Works

by Dr. Lia G. Andrews, DAOM, L.Ac.

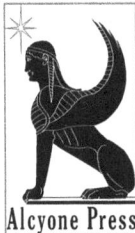

Alcyone Press

San Diego

Published by Alcyone Press
San Diego, CA
www.AlcyonePress.com

ISBN-10: 0989326063
ISBN-13: 978-0-9893260-6-3

This book is intended to be informational and should not be
considered a substitute for advice from a medical professional,
whom the reader should consult before beginning any diet or
exercise regimen, and before taking any dietary supplements or
other medications. The author and publisher expressly disclaim
responsibility for any adverse effects arising from the use or
application of the information in this book.

For information on Dr. Andrews' clinic in San Diego, please see
www.CinnabarAcupuncture.com

For rights and permission inquiries please contact the author
through her website: www.LiaAndrews.com

I Love My Body Series:
Book 1: I Love My Hormones; Understand & Balance Your 7 Year
Cycles
Book 2: I Love My Postpartum
Book 3: I Love My Period
Book 4: I Love My Skin; Natural Skincare That Actually Works
Book 5: I Love My Sensuality
Book 6: I Love My Menopase

Editors: Lia Andrews, Judith Andrews
Layout Design & Graphic Editing: PXPDesign.com
Cover Design: Lia Andrews
Author Photograph: Judith Andrews
Illustrations: Lia Andrews

Dedication

To Richard and Justin

Contents

Acknowledgements vii
Introduction ix

Overmedicated Skin 11

    Beauty as a Reflection of Health ... 13
    The Western Model 14
    What Most Products Do 17

Lifestyle for Healthy Skin 21

Nutrition for Radiant Skin 29

Supplements for Optimal Skin 39

    Supplements 39

Topical Products & Ingredients 45

    Actives 45
    Gentle Skin Repair 51
    Mineral Sunscreens 56
    Exfoliators 57
    Things to Remove From Your
    Skincare Regimen 59

Skincare Rituals 63

The Basic Skincare Ritual 64
The Youthing Ritual 67
The Skin Brightening Ritual 70
The Clear Skin Ritual 73
The Calming Ritual 79
Low Maintenance Rituals 82
Body Ritual 83
Resources 85
Skincare 85
Chinese Herbs 85
Chinese Ingredients 85
Credits 86
Index 87
About the Author 91

Acknowledgements

I want to thank Dr. Richard Huber and Justin Kovash from 302 Professional Skincare for their guidance and support in developing my skincare protocols and in writing this book.

I want to thank Miya Uchida of PXP Design for being a dear friend and teacher. She designed the inside of this book. Her ingenuity, work ethic, and attention to detail were necessary for the creation of this book. I want to thank my mom, Dr. Judith Andrews, for her constant support and technical insights.

Introduction

The I Love My Body Series of books and ebooks are short, action plans that focus on areas that most block our full expression, health, and empowerment.

I had health issues as a teenager that led me to seek alternative medical treatment, and eventually to become an acupuncturist. Part of that journey was my struggle with severe acne. I was on Accutane twice, took internal antibiotics for years, and was on every topical product, natural or prescription, ever marketed for acne (or at least that is how I felt). It took me a long time to heal my skin and to develop natural methods to help my patients.

My purpose in writing this book is to give people who committed to natural products and lifestyle a method to repair their skin and make it better than it has ever been. This book covers skincare for all ages.

Chapter 1

Overmedicated Skin

It took a bit of coaxing to pry my personal skincare arsenal of acids, benzoyl peroxide, and harsh detergents from my hands. After a decade battling severe acne I was finally forced to admit that I was addicted. And like every addiction, the harsh products simply offered a band-aid for a deeper problem.

Health problems led me to change my lifestyle and eventually become an acupuncturist. Though my acne improved as I became healthier, my skin was rough from years of harsh products and I still suffered from breakouts. I felt reliant upon constantly stripping my skin.

I was committed to living a natural, healthy lifestyle in every other area in my life, but the natural products and remedies I tried were ineffective at best, and more often made my skin worse. I tried the products at the health food

store or those I discovered from skincare forums.
I tried every home remedy, from oil washes to
apple cider vinegar to essential oil blends. They
would usually make my skin worse, sending me
back to harsh over-the-counter or prescription
products. These products would offer temporary
relief, but soon my skin would become flaky,
bumpy, and irritated and push me to search for
a natural alternative. I rode this roller coaster for
many years.

When I became an acupuncturist I was
determined to find a way to correct my skin
issues, and those of my patients, naturally. I used
everything I knew about cosmetic acupuncture,
Chinese herbal medicine, nutrition, lifestyle, as
well as experimented with countless products and
machines until I was finally able to create systems
that reliably produced results.

I am happy to report that I completely
transitioned to natural corrective skincare[1] six
years ago and will never go back. My skin is
healthy, resilient, and vibrant, and it stays this
way consistently. If I stop using products for a bit,
my skin stays healthy. In the next chapters I will
give you the methods I have developed, but first I
want to review some foundational concepts about
skincare and how products work.

---

1. The purpose of corrective skincare is to affect a change
in the skin.

Beauty as a Reflection of Health

We often hear that our skin is the biggest organ in our body. It is also the most visible. Our skin gives us an accurate window into what is going on internally. If our skin is saggy or thinning, so probably is our connective tissue throughout our body. If we have acne or rosacea, this points to internal toxicity and inflammation. Dark spots (hyperpigmentation) not only arise from sun exposure, but also from hormonal imbalance and sluggish lymphatic functioning.

In Traditional Chinese Medicine (TCM) there are two predominant models to describe skin aging. The first is *jing* depletion. *Jing* is the genetic and hormonal matter concentrated in our bone marrow, cerebral spinal fluid, endocrine organs, and brain that forms the foundation of our physical vitality.

The second model, is that with age *qi* (vital energy) becomes weaker and bodily processes become sluggish. There is a concurrent slowing in the microcirculation (*blood stasis*) and nutrients are unable to be properly distributed.

The Western Model

When we delve deep enough into TCM theory it meets with Western science's view of the skin. The phenotype lysyl oxidase is at the center of skin esthetics and moreover, our general health, as well as the Chinese concept of Jing. "To put it very technically: lysyl oxidase is a copper-dependent amine oxidase that oxidatively deaminates the peptidyl-lysine residues in collagen and elastin molecules and catalyses the formation of covalent cross-linkages of collagen or elastin which is necessary for the assembly of stable collagen and elastic fibers.

Another way to say that is that lysyl oxidase is the manufacturing director of the matrix we call our skin, indeed of our entire body in the form of the extracellular matrix. Lysyl oxidase is often referred to as LOXL and it may also be described as the software that directs the DNA to assemble fibers and just as importantly, to direct the signaling within the extracellular matrix where those fibers exist. LOXL may be the most essential epigenetic factor for quality of life."[2]

Anti-aging

Cross-linking and scar tissue formation = aging

---

2. Interview with Richard Huber (March 3, 2012).

"When LOXL performs well, we look and feel great. When we age poorly or undergo environmental stress (often the same thing), LOXL usually goes wrong. In its proper day-to-day work it knits together long ropes of fibers and maintains strong cellular architecture. However, this function can go askew and the knitting process, called crosslinking, results in many knots in the rope-like strands that displace natural moisture and cells begin to resemble cooked oatmeal dried in the sun. This happens inside and out by the way. Skin looks poorly textured and in time resembles one large, very thin sheet of scar tissue. In fact, scar tissue is formed by LOXL at wound sites. The purpose is to knit the body together quickly for protection. Aged skin does not have to become a thin sheet of gristle, however. The key is to strongly limit stressing the skin with harsh chemicals like exfoliating acids or benzoyl peroxide or too much of even ordinary topical products and of course, too much direct sunlight. One last thing to know – sunscreens won't prevent LOXL from going wrong."[3]

Hyperpigmentation (Dark Spots, Cholasma)

Cells trapped in cross linking = hyperpigmentation

"As we age, or put our skin under stress, other

---

3. Interview with Richard Huber (March 3, 2012).

dysfunctions occur, especially the breakdown of the waste product removal process in the skin. In addition, during hormonal stress, or even pregnancy, pigmentation cells can arise as a mechanism by the skin immune process. The combination of a breakdown in normal functions and an increase in pigment cells can lead to a very uneven look to the skin. This collection of cell waste product, called lipofuscin, and excess pigment cells that normally would be sloughed off the skin surface, or be routed to the lymphatic 'drains' in the dermis, instead can be caught in the skin as LOXL wraps the waste in a fibrotic cocoon or gristle. And there it all sits as the skin becomes ever thinner and loses its functionality. Spots, texture problems, uneven tone, and thin, blah skin results. To correct this, LOXL must be normalized and the gristle softened and the waste moved out of the skin. The situation is not so dark, however. There are now noninvasive, inexpensive and simple esthetic procedures and products to effect that desired result."[4]

Acne (Inflammation)

Crazy cell proliferation = acne

"Most of the difficulties from acne originate with a surge in total cell numbers without an equal surge in the removal of old cells. It is skin, literally

---

4. Interview with Richard Huber (March 3, 2012).

out of balance. This proliferation of cells leads to crowding and a loss of skin architecture and dysfunction processes get underway. Here, LOXL has a role in reacting to a surge in hormones by doing a great job of producing huge quantities of unwanted skin cells that can pour out like lava from a volcano. In this situation, the skin begins to look thick, uneven in texture and can be pitted and at the end of the ordeal may now be scarred. This fibrotic mass of skin can aggravate more acne formation and now a vicious circle is in play. LOXL normalized will lead to normal sebaceous gland output and reduce acne significantly as well as reduce the fibrotic mass. There are fortunately simple, non-prescription techniques and products today to normalize skin functions and eliminate the scars and excess cell production associated with acne."[5]

What Most Products Do

The vast majority of skincare products and treatments do not come close to affecting lysyl oxidase functioning. Many products that offer "instant" results such as plumping up fine lines, minimizing pores, or firming the skin do so by creating temporary inflammation. Once the inflammation goes down the results disappear. Relying on products that strip the skin or cause

5. Interview with Richard Huber (March 3, 2012).

inflammation can cause permanent damage over time.

In optimizing the condition of our skin we want to take full advantage of internal and external methods available to us. In the next chapters we will work from the inside out.

DISCLAIMER:

I am a an unabashed fan of 302 Professional Skincare. I use their product line as the core of my topical skincare approach, and other natural products supplementally. If you want to use other products you can follow the same principles presented here and apply them.

Chapter 2

Lifestyle for Healthy Skin

Internal health is the foundation for healthy skin. It all begins with the decisions we make on a daily basis.

Sleep

A teacher of mine used to say that not getting to bed before 10 each night "makes you stupid." Perhaps this is the blunt Chinese way to motivate people. Inadequate sleep will not only adversely affect brain functioning, it also causes premature aging and weight gain. The hours between 10 p.m. and midnight are the most restorative hours of sleep. It is best to retire when you feel a little tired, as going to bed exhausted weakens the kidneys and adrenals. Make sure to get 8-9 hours of uninterrupted sleep each night. Also, go to bed and wake up with a smile. Another teacher of mine firmly believes this is the key to staying young.

Regular Relaxation

Emotional stress is the single biggest factor in pathology and premature aging. Learning to calm your mind and emotions is the most important step to retaining your youth and vitality and achieving long life. Most of life is outside our control and this naturally produces stress. Stress does not help us. Rather it scatters and disconnects us from ourselves by placing the focus on the chaos of the world. We can only begin to take control of our minds and emotions when we accept that the only thing we have control over is how we respond to life. We must make a daily commitment to practice relaxation techniques and to let go of negative events and people. When we feel overwhelmed, we must seek out friends to talk with or healers to help us relax.

Exercise 2.1. Grace Prayer

This is my modification of Thich Nhat Hanh's Meditation Poem.[1] Use it throughout the day to

---

1. Thich Nhat Hanh, *The Heart of the Buddha's Teaching; Transforming Suffering into Peace, Joy, and Liberation.* (Berkeley: Parallax Press,1998).

stay connected or in seated meditation. Speak the words to yourself in your mind, not out loud.

1. "In" (inhale)
2. "Out" (exhale)
3. "Deep" (inhale)
4. "Slow" (exhale)
5. "Kindness" (inhale)
6. "Grace" (exhale)
7. "Beautiful Moment" (inhale)
8. "Present Moment" (exhale)

Balanced Work

Overworking mentally, especially when straining on a computer, taxes our *yin*[2] energy and unbalances our livers. Overworking physically, depletes our *yang*[3] energy. Even if you are still young enough to test your physical limits, one day the reserves simply will not be there anymore. It is better never to reach this day. Overworking to collapse is a sure way to chronic fatigue syndrome and fibromyalgia. Rather, balance periods of overexertion with periods of rest.

---

2. *Yin* is a fundamental concept in Daoism and Chinese medicine. In terms of the body, *yin* is associated with substance, abundance of fluids, suppleness, elasticity, and flexibility.

3. *Yang* is a fundamental concept in Daoism and Chinese medicine. In terms of the body, *yang* is associated with action, organ and cellular functioning, heat, and generation of power.

Exercises that Balance

Maintaining youthfulness for life requires a shift from recklessness to awareness. You cannot make your body more beautiful while you mistreat yourself. The mark of a good exercise routine is that your body moves better and has more vitality. Healthy exercise supports microcirculation and lymphatic flow. As always, by increasing our internal health, we are promoting the beauty of our skin.

Exercise 2.2. Rules for Exercise

1. Warm up your joints prior to exercising with mobility drills. Finish your workout routines with stretching. These steps protect against injury and increase neuroconnections in the body.
2. Limit cardio to 45 min. Excessive cardio depletes your body and does more harm than good. If you enjoy running, do short 45-sec. sprints between walking.
3. Lift heavy weights 3 times a week, giving yourself ample rest in between. This builds muscle, strengthens bones and ligaments, and promotes fat loss.
4. Try to exercise between sunrise and sunset. This is *yang* time when you should naturally be active. When the sun

has set, *yin* grows strong and it is time for rest.

5. Do not go to exhaustion. The ideal time to stop is when you feel energetic and alive. This will produce better aesthetic and health results.

6. If you have dry skin or suffer heat signs (such as acne, rosacea, or hot flashes) avoid hot yoga and limit saunas until the condition is stabilized. These will increase heat and dry up the body, maing them ideal for those who run cold and suffer from phlegm or excess weight.

Self-Concept

Confidence

It is hard to feel confident when we suffer from a skin condition, especially when it is on our face. The learning experience we can gain from this is to know our own worth despite the (perceived or real) judgements of others. We can also look beyond the cosmetic façade of others and see them as they are. Your condition is temporary. With the tools in this book and perhaps the guidance of esthetic and health professionals you will emerge with beautiful skin, and hopefully a little wisdom.

Youthfulness

Actress Sophia Loren once said that the secret

to her youthfulness was she kept perfect posture and she did not "make old people noises." What starts the process of aging is that we begin to think, feel, and act old. It is the expectation that by such and such age "I will be old." If we ignore the common level of consciousness, we will live a different reality. Have the expectation that you will live with vitality for the rest of your life; that rather than closing in on you, life will continue to expand.

See yourself as beautiful and healthy and take actions to affirm this daily. This becomes more important over the years because there is increasing social pressure to start behaving like an old person. Keep yourself manicured at all times, as if you were going to meet a new lover. Wear pretty underwear. Adorn yourself with clothes, accessories, and scents that make you feel beautiful.

This is not the same, however, as behaving childishly or dressing inappropriately. Wisdom and grace are natural gifts we acquire from living longer. We can integrate these while keeping up our curiosity, passion, and energy.

Next we will cover another foundation for healthy skin; nutrition.

Chapter 3

Nutrition for Radiant Skin

It is one of the most oft spoken lies about skin health that it is not affected by your diet. An unbalanced diet can cause or aggravate acne, rosacea, dryness, oiliness, wrinkles, dull complexion, etc. While a healthy diet will help make the most of your genetics.

General Dietary Rules for Healthy Skin

1. **Drink adequate water**. Adequate hydration helps our bodies excrete toxins and aids in virtually all of our bodies' functioning. Dehydration can cause constipation, dry skin, stubborn weight gain, and give a deflated look to our skin. Be sure to avoid drinking water 30 minutes before or after meals as it dilutes digestive enzymes. It is a good practce to drink an 8 ounce glass

of warm water first think in the morning to promote bowel regularity. An easy calculation to estimate adequate water intake is:

weight in lbs. x 2/3 = ____ ounces

2. **Eat a balance of protein, healthy fats, complex carbohydrates, and low glycemic vegetables**. In Chinese medicine each of these groups has a vital function that balances the others. Protein builds the body. Healthy fats lubricate the body. Complex carbohydrates provide energy. Vegetables cool and cleanse. Fruit also has a cooling and cleansing action, but high sugar content can be destabilizing in a diet already high in sugars.

3. **Eat every 4 hours**. Eating smaller meals throughout the day helps boost metabolism and keeps blood sugar levels stable. Unstable blood sugar can trigger inflammatory skin conditions such as acne.

4. **Limit sugar intake**. Sweets should be an ocassional treat. Excessive sugar intake destabilizes blood sugar and is a primary aggravator of acneic conditions.

Top 9 Chinese Superfoods

Additionally, there are foods we can eat regularly for their anti-aging qualities. They enhance brain function, beautify the skin, boost the hormones, and promote longevity. These foods appear regularly in Chinese Food Therapy. They also help protect against deficiency in vegetarians or those who want to reduce meat intake.[1]

Longan berries, go ji berries, and mullberries are potent superfoods that can (and should) be eaten indefinitely without creating imbalances.

1. **Longan Berries** – are very high in iron and beautify the skin. They aid cognitive functioning, calm anxiety, and help build the blood. Longan berries are ideal for students or those who do a great deal of mental work. They are excellent for the elderly, those recovering from illness or emotional trauma, and postpartum or post-menstral women. Eat them for symptoms such as weakness, insomnia, worry, forgetfulness, and palpitations. Eat them fresh or dried in soups, congee, smoothies, trail mix, etc.

2. **Go Ji Berries** – are an ideal general antiaging herb. They beautify the skin and hair. Go ji berries are excellent for

---

1. Sun Simiao specifically noted that cow's milk, black sesame seeds, and bee honey were "far better than meats."

symptoms of blurry vision, weakness of low back and knees, premature gray hair, infertility, dry cough, and inflamed prostate. They can stimulate contraction of the uterus and should be used with caution during fragile pregnancies, but are ideal for postpartum and during menses. Eat them fresh or dried in soups, congee, smoothies, trail mix, etc.

3. **Mulberries** – beautify the skin and lubricate the bowels to treat constipation. They are used for symptoms of dizziness, blurred vision, premature gray hair, hot flashes, weakness of low back and knees, tinnitus, and insomnia. Mulberries are an excellent long-term tonic for women who are depleted by their monthly periods. Eat them fresh or dried in soups, congee, smoothies, trail mix, etc.

4. **Black Sesame Seeds** – lubricate the bowels for constipation. They are used for premature gray hair, insufficient milk in nursing mothers, blurred vision, and tinnitus. Brown sesame seeds go to the Spleen and also lubricate the intestines to treat constipation, but do not have the same antiaging power that black sesame seeds do. Grind and use in soups, congee, smoothies, etc.

5. **Jujube Dates** – boost energy, build

the blood, calm the emotions, and protect the liver against toxins. (For this reason they are recommended prior to and after surgery). They are used for fatigue, pallor, low appetite, muscle weakness, scanty menses, blurred vision, irritability, and emotional instability resulting in hysterical crying. Avoid in cases of yeast infection or intestinal parasites. Eat them fresh or dried in soups, congee, smoothies, baking, etc.

6. **Mushrooms** – There are numerous types of mushrooms that are useful in regular diet to prevent disease as they concurrently tonify deficiencies and clear excesses. Mushrooms in general conteract the heavy nature of a high protein diet and strengthen the immune system. **Black wood ear mushroom** hydrates the body and moistens the skin. It is used to promote blood circulation and dispell fluid accumulation. **White cloud mushroom** moistens and beautifies the skin.

7. **Bee Products** – **Honey** detoxifies the body and harmonizes the liver. It is useful in the overworked, menstrual disorders, excess rich foods, constipation, stomach ulcers. Pasteurized or heat-processed honey moistens the body. Raw honey (comb

honey) drys fluid accumulations (edema, excess weight, and phlegm conditions). Raw honey contains pollen and all of its properties.[2] **Local bee pollen** is excellent for treating allergies and building immunity. For this purpose take regularly and continuously. For allergies take 1 tsp daily. For athletic endurance take 2-3 tsp daily. It decreases the need for animal proteins. **Bee Propolis** is a natural antiseptic that kills bacteria, fungus, and viruses. It is used for toxins in the body. Propolis is a resinous substance bees use to seal small holes and cracks in the structure of the hive. It helps to strengthen the hive and ward off diseases that could attack in the crowded beehive workspace. **Royal Jelly** is a powerful rejuvenation tonic for both men and women. It decreases the need for animal proteins and is used to increase fertility.[3]

8. **Collagen-rich foods** – Ingest collagen-rich foods daily to rejuvenate the skin

---

2. Paul Pitchford. *Healing With Whole Foods; Oriental Traditions and Modern Nutrition.* (Berkeley: North Atlantic Books, 1993), 151.

3. There have always been stories about beekeepers living long healthy lives which were attributed to the properties of the pollen, honey, royal jelly, or propolis. My experience is that these longevity benefits are in fact due to the process of keeping bees. To keep bees successfully and naturally requires being intune with the cycles of nature, calming the emotions in their presence, and being in service to the tiniest of creatures.

and joints. The best foods are bone broth made with connective tissue, gelatin, and chicken feet or pork trotters. Collagen supplements can be taken instead.

9. **The 5 Beans** – Different types of beans pertain to the different elements and should be eaten regularly to balance the major organ systems. **Mung Beans** detoxify the liver and gallbladder systems and clear toxicity from the body. **Lima Beans** nourish the lungs and beautify the skin. **Red Adzuki Beans** reduce edema and support heart functioning. **Black Beans** tonify the kidneys. **Soybeans** support the spleen.

Wrinkles & Dry Skin

Our skin tends to become drier as we age. In Chinese medicine this is because *yin*[(4)] declines over time. In Western terms, sex hormone levels that preserve the skin become depleted. Dry weather, blood deficiency, medication, or genetics can also cause dry skin. Wrinkles occur when there are a lack of nutrients and energy to the surface of the skin.

To internally plump up the skin the first step is to drink ample water. You should also eat hydrating

---

4. *Yin* is a fundamental concept in Daoism and Chinese medicine. In terms of the body, *yin* is associated with abundance of fluids, suppleness, elasticity, and flexibility.

foods such as soups, broths, and smoothies. **Include** healthy fats such as avocado, nuts and seeds, cocoa butter, olive oil, and coconut oil, though in moderation as these are difficult to digest. Healthy dairy products such as kefir and yogurt are also moistening as long as they do not cause phlegm. Other foods that moisten the skin include mulberries, pears, and white cloud mushroom. Unrefined salt with a balanced mineral profile helps your body retain hydration.

Acne

Acne always involves heat (inflammation), which may be caused by hormonal or digestive imbalances, stress, or other reasons. Women in their 30s and 40s often develop acne on the chin or jawline, which relates to hormonal imbalance.

Make sure to optimize bowel movements, as even minor constipation will increase heat and toxicity in the body. Drink plenty of water between meals and eat vegetables at every meal. **Include** mung beans, dandelion and other bitter greens, milk thistle tincture, probiotics, and seaweed (or kelp pills) daily in the diet. **Avoid** heating or inflammatory substances: sugar, spices, garlic, alcohol, and marijuana. Dairy and food sensitivities can trigger breakouts in some individuals.

Hyperpigmentation (Dark Spots, Sun Spots, Cholasma)

Hyperpigmentation occurs more frequently in those with higher melanin production. The more you tan and the less you burn in the sun, the more predisposed you are to dark spots as you age. Living in a dry, sunny climate also increases hyperpigmentation. Asians, Latinos, and lighter complexion African Americans are particularly susceptible. Hyperpigmentation occurs when the dermis is injured, as an inflammatory reaction, sun damage, and due to hormonal fluctuations (as occurs during pregnancy). When treating ark spots, avoid sun exposure as much as possible and use an SPF of 30 or more.

When treating the body internally for dark spots, the key is to balance the liver. Take milk thistle tincture daily, along with pearl powder and Avogen™. Eat foods high in vitamin C such as citrus, green leafy vegetables broccoli, berries, tomatoes, peas, and papaya.

In the next chapter we will cover supplementation.

Chapter 4

Supplements for Optimal Skin

Proper supplements build on a healthy diet and lifestyle. They protect us against the inevitable times when we do not get enough sleep, or are stressed out, or do not have access to healthy food. These are a list of supplements I find most important for optimum skin health. Customized herbal formulas from a licensed herbalist are also highly effective to treat specific skin conditions.

Supplements

Avocatin 302 / Avogen™

Avogen™ is the most important internal beauty supplement, that has far reaching health benefits as well. It is a matrix of small molecules extracted from specific species of avocado. Avogen™ was discovered by Dr. Richard Huber on an expedition to Guatemala where he noticed that one particular group of locals displayed no sun damage, despite the high altitude and harsh sun exposure. Whereas their neighbors showed expected signs of wrinkles, sagging, and dark spots as they aged. He observed that the unaged group would make a cooked gruel of small local avocadoes, and ate it as a staple every morning. This was the hint that led Dr. Huber to eventually isolate and patent the responsible compound; Avocatin 302. Avogen™ is the internal product containing Avocatin 302. It preserves skin suppleness and thickness, and treats dark spots (hyperpigmentation) and scarring. It is even effective for pitting acne scars when taken daily for 9-12 months.

What Avogen™ does for the surface of the skin, it also does internally. It strengthens the integrity of connective tissue and our "inner skin." It breaks up old adhesions and scar tissue and disinhibits the formation of new scar tissue, making invaluable for those with old or recent surgeries and injuries. If you use Avogen™ daily you will notice that it speeds skin cell turnover as well as hair and nail growth, though it does not thicken hair and nails. It will thicken the epidermis and is effective for thinning skin. Recent studies have even shown it effective against certain types of cancer.

Avocatin 302 is found in varying amounts in different species and crops of avocadoes and is often concentrated in the seed. Heat makes Avocatin 302 more bio-available. Thus, you would not only need to eat 1 cooked avocado per day to equal 1 capsule of Avogen™, it would also have to be the right species. (Avocadoes are excellent in the diet, especially for those with dry skin or who are losing plumpness in their skin.)

Collagen

Collagen is a protein and a building block of our skin. As we age, collagen production decreases. Collagen supplementation is helpful as part of an antiaging program and to strengthen the joints. This is why in Asian cultures you will often see women eating chicken feet or pork trotters, which are natural sources of collagen.

Keratin

Keratin is another protein present in the body that aids n the repair of skin, hair, and nails.

Multivitamin

A good general multivitamin helps ensure that we get adequate vital nutrients if they are absent from our diet on a day to day basis. **Vitamin A** is essential for skin health and repair. It helps treat wrinkles and acne, just as topical application does. **Biotin** is a building block of skin, hair, and nails. Supplementation often provides visible changes in the vibrancy of hair. **Vitamin C** protects your skin from sun damage, just as topical application does. It also aids in skin repair. **Vitamin E** protects against sun damage and helps prevent wrinkles. **Zinc** aids in wound repair, regulates the release of vitamin A, and can be used to help control acne. **Selenium** is an antioxidant that can aid the treatment of acne.

Omega 3 Fatty Acids

These oils are found in cold water fish, flaxseeds, and safflower oil. The modern American diet often does not provide adequate amounts. Omega 3 supplementation can be helplful in inflammatory skin conditions such as acne and dry skin.

Kelp (Kombu Seaweed)

Seaweed cools inflammation, drains edema, and softens masses. It is helpful in many acneic or inflammatory skin conditions. Kelp is considered the strongest and is most often used in herbal medicine.

Pearl Powder

Pearl powder is an ancient treatment and preventive for freckles, liver spots, cholasma, and general hyperpigmentation. Pearl powder clears acne, eczema, and non-healing sores. In addition to beautifying the skin, pearl powder calms the emotions and treats palpitations, insomnia, visual disturbances, eye disorders, and tension.

Milk Thistle Tincture

Milk thistle detoxifies and protects the liver. Clearing toxins from the bodies promotes clear, vibrant skin. Take away from medication and supplements as milk thistle has a flushing action on the liver and can inhibit absorption when taken together.

In the next chapter we will move to the external and discuss what you put on your skin.

Chapter 5
Topical Products & Ingredients

Actives

Actives are topicals that function like medicine. You use them with a specific dosage and frequency to treat a concern. Too little will be ineffective, while excessive use can cause side effects. In terms of actives, the most common side effect is topical irritation. Actives are the most important players in a corrective skincare plan, but they must be treated with respect.

Avocatin 302 / Avogen™
This is my favorite skincare ingredient due to its high efficacy and minimal side effects. It is extracted from a specific strain of avocados. As skin ages it begins to form excessive cross-linking which asphyxiates the cells, becoming more like scar tissue. Avocatin 302 undoes this excessive cross-linking. I recommend using it internally as

well as externally to preserve the health of your skin and treating most skin conditions.

Dr. Richard Huber, who first discovered and utilized this compound, calls avocatin 302 "a unique product of the rainforest discovered on a botanical research expedition into Central America. Found nowhere else in nature, this skin active matrix developed in an isolated species of avocado and plays the key role in the folklore of the fruit and its benefits to the skin. When applied topically, Avocatin 302 builds skin protein in the epidermis and dermis which may have thinned or become heavy and inelastic because of age or the environment. Structurally, it is a lipid that contains a matrix of small molecules which have a marked affinity for skin enzymes that regulate skin metabolism, especially as we age. These are low molecular weight, high electron content substances with an array metabolites for the skin and more generally for the entire extra cellular matrix itself."[1]

The 302 molecule:
- increases the energy in the skin
- increases circulation to the skin
- softens the skin

---

1. 302 Professional Skincare Quick Reference Guide.

WARNING:

302 Professional Skincare products that contain the 302 matrix are not compatible with home care products containing exfoliating acids, such as lactic, glycolic, malic, azaleic and others, nor with phenols like salicylic acid. If you use acids in your homecare, use the commercially available Avogen™Avocado Topical Mist. Avogen™ Avocado Dietary Supplement can be taken internally without any problems. If you get a professional peel and use a professional product containg 302, stop using it until your skin has healed. Also note that using the 302 matrix on your skin will make your skin more active and it might react stronger to a peel. All other 302 Professional Skincare products may be used with exfoliating acids.

- works synergistically to improve the efficacy of other actives
- normalizes skin cell production
- calms irritation
- thickens the epidermis
- generally rejuvenate the skin without causing side effects

Products:
Avogen™ Avocado Topical Mist (less concentrated), 302 Plus Drops or Serum (medium concentration), 302 Sensitive Drops (medium concentration), 302 Drops

or Serum (high concentration). Small amounts present in 302 Cleanser, 302 Face & Body Bar, and 302 Body Treatment: Intensive.

Vitamin A

Vitamin A is a highly versatile ingredient that weeds out defective or excessive cells and helps build healthy ones. It is powerful and effective against acne, wrinkles, hyperpigmentation, and loss of tone when used sparingly. Retinyl acetate, retinyl palmitate, retinol, and retinaldehyde are all forms of vitamin A that the skin converts to retinoic acid. Retinoic acid is the active form that reacts with the skin.[2]

Vitamin A:

- increases healthy cell growth
- generates new capillary growth
- improves protein deposition in the epidermis
- helps control pigmentation problems
- rebuilds thin weak skin
- helps reduce wrinkles
- reduces acne breakouts

There are a number of cautions and contraindications for using vitamin A. Retinyl acetate and palmitate are less

2. Retinoic acid is only available by medical prescription. It is stronger but also highly irritating when applied topically.

phototoxic than other vitamin A forms, but it is still important to stay out of the sun after applying. Apply at night and wash off in the morning. Most people achieve best results when using vitamin A 1-3 times per week. When used too frequently, it causes redness, dryness, and irritation when used excessively. Overuse can cause sensitization. Contraindicated during pregnancy and nursing.

Products:
302 A-Boost (contains retinyl palmitate),
302 Clarity (contains retinyl acetate)

Vitamin C - tetrahexydecylascorbate (THDCA)[3]

Vitamin C is highly effective in the treatment of dark spots (hyperpigmentation), thin weak skin, and sun damage. It also protects the skin against future damage. Most products use ascorbic acid; a water-soluble form of vitamin C. Ascorbic acid oxidizes and rapidly becomes ineffective when exposed to oxygen.[4] THDCA is an oil-soluble form of Vitamin C that remains active on the skin for 48

---

3. Google "BV-OSC" to read human study results in a study using C-Boost concentrations of THDCA.

4. This is why many vitamin C products turn brown. It means the vitamin C has oxidied and no longer has a therapeutic effect.

hours (meaning it only needs to be applied every other day) and has a long shelf-life.

Vitamin C:
- thickens the dermis
- brightens the skin
- protects against sun damage and free radicals[5]

Excessive use stops producing results, but other vitamn C tends to be well tolerated.

Products:
302 Plus Drops or Serum (less concentrated), 302 C-Boost (medium concentration), 302 Lightening Drops (high concentration)

Niacinamide - Vitamin B3

Niacinamide causes a surge in circulation to the surface of the skin. It promotes the absorption of other skincare ingredients and is particularly useful for non-responsive or aged skin.

- increases cellular energy
- improves cell metabolism
- increases capillary formation

---

5. Smoking (tobacco and marijuana) leeches vitamin C from the skin. If you smoke be sure to add viamin C to your regimen.

- decreases the look of dark under eye
  circles

Avoid in cases of inflamed skin, such as
acne or rosacea.

Products:
302 Plus Drops and Serum, 302 Eye
Firming Serum

Peptides

Peptides can be derived from various
natural sources. They increase moisture and
have a plumping action on the skin.

Products:
302 Plus Drops and Serum, 302 Eye
Firming Serum

Gentle Skin Repair

Many skin concerns originate from inflammation
and bacteria. These topical ingredients help
protect and repair the skin.

Zinc Oxide

Besides being an excellent sunscreen,
zinc oxide soothes inflammation, is
antibacterial, and aids wound healing. It is
a key ingredient in treating inflammatory

conditions such as rosacea, acne, or irritate skin.

Product:
302 Remedy Rx

Concentrated ECGC in Green Tea

Green tea has long been used for its soothing and antibacterial properties, however the active compound, ECGC (epigallocatechin), is often found in proximity to the caffeine molecule, which can be damaging to the skin with regular use. By isolating the ECGC from green tea you get the benefits without the side effects.

Product:
302 Calming Mist

Ammonia Polymer

Ammonia (NH4) is not your traditional "natural" remedy, but it does have a long unofficial tradition by Russian beauties in their homecare regimens. Properly extracted from natural sources, ammonia polymer is a highly effective soothing, antibacterial, and anti-inflammatory topical agent, powerful enough to replace benzoyl peroxide in your homecare regimen, without any of the side effects.

The way it works is that ammonia is an

active precursor of carbamide phosphate, which is an essential component of protein synthesis in the skin. It can be used to treat acne, dry aged skin, and nervy conditions such as shingles. It is stinky for a moment until it drys and should be used in a well ventilated area. **Be sure not to avoid the eye area.**

Product:
302 Revive Rx

Sulfur

Sulfur is antibacterial and anti-inflammatory when applied topically. It has been used cross-culturally, in both traditional and modern medicines, as an effective treatment for acne, dermatitis, rosacea, and eczema. Excessive use can be drying.

Product:
302 Acne Cleanser Rx, 302 Treatment Mask

Colloidal Silver[6]

Used in Western medicine to combat bacterial infections prior to the widespread availability of antibiotics. Topically, it soothes inflammation, is antibacterial, and

6. Much has been made about the dangers of colloidal silver and its ability to turn people's skin blue. Argyria, the medical name for this condition, occurs from excessive and longterm internal ingestion of colloidal silver.

aids wound healing. A great remedy for burned, irritated, or wounded skin is to saturate gauze in colloidal silver and apply it as a compress for 10 minutes, twice daily.

Product:
Available at health food stores

Hydrators

Natural moisturizers can be used as needed to keep the skin hydrated and supple. A good hydrator helps to build up the skin barrier leaving the skin more resilient and does not cause dependency. Keep your moisturizers as a separate product and avoid ones that contain retinols or other actives as they invariably lead to over-usage of those actives.

Jojoba Oil

An oil extracted from the seed of the jojoba shrub, native to the American southwest and Mexico. It is easily absorbed into the skin, well tolerated by most skin types, and has a long shelf-life.

Products:
302 Moisturizing Drops, all 302 lipid-based products, 302 Recovery Plus, 302 Recovery Plus: Intensive, 302 Day/Night

Refined Coconut Oil

Oil extracted from coconuts. The unrefined oil is excellent for cooking and protects the hair when applied topically, but can cause breakouts when applied to the skin. The refined oil is a staple in skin care.

Products:
302 Moisturizing Drops, all 302 lipid-based products

Refined Avocado Oil

An oil extracted from the pulp of avocados. The unrefined version is edible, but can case breakouts when applied topically. Refined avocado oil is emolliating and rejuvenates the skin when applied.

Products:
302 Moisturizing Drops, all 302 lipid-based products, 302 Recovery Plus, 302 Recovery Plus: Intensive, 302 Day/Night

Cocoa Butter

A fat extracted from the cocoa bean native to the Amazon. It is used in chocolate production, and also to thicken creams and ointments. Cocoa butter imparts a chocolate smell.

Products:
302 Recovery Plus, 302 Recovery Plus:
Intensive, 302 Day/Night

Shea Butter
A thick fat extracted from the nut of the
shea tree that grows in parts of Africa. It
has been used for millenia to thicken
creams and ointments and to protect skin
and hair dry weather and harsh sun. It is
also used in cooking.

Product:
302 Day/Night

Mineral Sunscreens

Mineral sunscreens sit on the surface of the
skin and reflect back the sun's rays. They do
not penetrate or irritate the skin like chemical
sunscreens do, nor do they put off those funny
chemical odors. When you look on the "active
ingredients" on the back of sunscreen it should list
both titanium dioxide and zinc oxide and nothing
else. This combination will provide full UV-A and
UV-B protection. Apply in the morning as the
final step of your skin ritual prior to leaving the
house.

Products:
302 SPF-15, 30, & 50, 302 Recovery
Minerals (SPF-30)

Zinc Oxide

A natural mineral that not only reflects
ultraviolet radiation, but also promotes
wound healing and calms irritation
and redness. It can be drying when
used to excess. Safe particle sizes are
> 100 ug. Smaller particles, often called
micronized zinc, can interfere with cellular
metabolism.[7]

Titanium Dioxide

Another natural mineral that reflects
ultraviolet radiation. Again, be sure to use
in safe particle sizes > 100 ug, in order to
avoid interference with cellular metabolism.

Exfoliators

Enzymes

Enzymatic exfoliation is more gentle and
less likely to cause irritation. It is safe for
more frequent use than acid or mechanical

7. Zinc and titanium provide a physical barrier to the
sun, and they often leave a pasty white color to the skin,
prompting many sunscreen manufacturers to use smaller
less visible particles. Smaller particles, however, can
potentially be absorbed by the skin, causing irritation and
toxicity. Instead, choose mineral sunscreens or powders
that have a tint that match your skin tone.

exfoliation (such as microdermabrasion). Occasional exfoliation is helpful to remove dead cells, and is useful in the treatment of rough skin or acne. **Bromelain enzyme** is a naturally ocurring enzyme derived from pineapple that exfoliates while reducing inflammation. Another enzyme popular in skincare is **papain**, a digestive enzyme derived from papaya that breaks down protein. It is very effective to remove dead skin cells without exfoliating healthy live cells.

Products:
302 Enzyme Mist

Acids

All acids: alpha hydroxy acids (AHAs), natural fruit acids, lactic acid, glycolic acid, salicylic acid, etc. should be used sparingly. I recommend they only be used in professional treatments and not in homecare regimens. Timed correctly they are effective in addressing conditions such as acne and dark spots (hyperpigmentation). With excessive use over time, acids weaken the skin and cause iritation; pre-aging the skin.

Salicylic acid (carboxyphenol) is often called a beta hydroxy acid, differentiated from alpha hydroxy acids by its lipophylic nature. It is in fact not a true acid, but a phenol. It has anti-inflammatory properties and eats up non-functioning cells in the epidermis. It is safer than other acids, but should still be used sparingly in professional treatments.

Things to Remove From Your Skincare Regimen

Benzoyl Peroxide

Benzoyl peroxide is a potent free radical creator. It tends to offer fast results in acne cases, but quickly the skin becomes rough, dry, and irritated, followed by a more virulent resurgence of breakouts. Regular use can destroy the skin longterm, and many skincare experts recommend limiting use to 3 months at a stretch. There are safer alternatives.

Replace With:
302 Revive Rx

Chemical Sunscreens

Unlike mineral sunblocks that sit on the surface of the skin like a shield, chemical sunscreens are absorbed and interact chemically with the skin. This is why they must be applied 30 minutes prior to sun exposure and need to be re-applied every 2 hours. Several chemical sunscreen ingredients are known carcinogens and they tend to irritate the skin. Many skincare experts are finding that they can cause more damage to the skin than the sun.

Replace With:
302 sunscreens, mineral make-up powders, or other mineral-based sunscreens.

Detergents (Sulfates)

Sudsy cleansers contain harsh detergents that strip and irritate the skin.

Replace With:
All 302 cleansers are detergent free.

Finally, in the next chapter we will cover skincare rituals to transform your skin.

Chapter 6

Skincare Rituals

With all the internal care, an effective skincare ritual is still necessary to bring out the most in your skin. Proper skincare helps prevent damage and slows the speed at which your skin shows aging.

Principles of Good Skincare:

1. **Less is More** - As women we are often trained to overdo it. We feel we must constantly be doing or applying something. Though this attitude helps fuel the commercial economy, skincare OCD is not good for the longterm health of our skin. This does not mean we should neglect our skin. Rather, using effective products and treatments at proper intervals will extend the vitality of our skin, as well as our pocket books.

2. **Exercise Your Skin Regularly** - Like everything in the human body, regular, non-damaging stimulation keeps things functioning optimally. This means

1. getting treatments like lymphatic drainage and facial massage or using active ingredients listed in the previous chapter.
2. **Minimize Make-Up** - If your goal is longterm healthy skin you should minimize the amount of makeup you wear. Healthy skin requires minimal coverage. Be sure to remove any make-up thoroughly each night before bed. This is ideally done with an oil-based cleanser. In Japan, women typically cleanse twice, first with oil to remove make-up and pollutants, and second with a soapy cleanser. You can use pure jojoba oil or a Japanese oil wash such as Noriko Cleansing Oil. Another choice is to use an oil-rich cleanser such as 302 Normal/Dry Cleanser.

The Basic Skincare Ritual

The best treatment is prevention. This ritual is ideal for those without skin issues.

Morning:

Cleansing

The skin should be cleansed 1-2 times a day. The morning requires only a quick, light cleanse or a rinse with cool water. 302 Face & Body Bar is a good choice.

Hydration

Apply a little 302 Eye Firming Serum around the eyes. Apply a moisturizer if your skin feels dry. If light moisturization is required, use 302 Recovery Plus. For normal to dry skin, choose between 302 Recovery Plus: Intensive or 302 Day/Night (lotions), or 302 Moisturizing Drops (oil).

Sun Protection

Mineral sunblock is critical to protect against premature aging. A sunscreen with a 30 SPF is preferable for daily use. If you are out in the elements, hiking or swimming, a 50 SPF is ideal.

You can combine sun protection and light coverage make-up. For a drier finish use a natural mineral makeup powder or 302 Recovery Minerals (SPF-30). For a more dewy finish, apply 1 pump of 302 Moisturizing Drops, mist with Calming Mist, then apply a thin layer of 302 SPF-30: Tinted.

Evening:

Cleansing

The evening requires more thorough

cleansing to remove dirt, pollutants, and make-up. You will wash twice. Apply a dime-size amount of 302 Cleanser (lotion) with dry fingers on dry skin. Massage into the skin to bind to impurities. Then wet your fingers and apply another dime-size amount, massaging into your skin. Rinse thoroughly until there is no more slick.

If your skin is oily, add lather from 302 Face & Body Bar prior to rinsing.

If you wear make-up, use 302 Normal/ Dry Cleanser in the same manner as 302 Cleanser.

Actives

Even when there are no skin issues, it is a good idea to apply key actives in lower concentrations once a week, on separate evenings. Most women do best on 302 A-Boost (Vitamin A), 302 C-Boost (Vitamin C), and 302 Drops.[1] To apply, mist the face with 302 Calming Mist, then apply 1 pump to the entire face, neck, and décolleté, wiping residual oil on the hands. Besides the three evenings in which you apply an active, you can simply apply a moisturizer as needed.

---

1. Do not use any products containing the 302 molecule, such as 302 Drops, if you are using any products with acids listed as an ingredient.

Hydration

Hydration that does not cause dependency or clog pores is an important part of skincare, especially in drier climates. If your skin is normal to oily apply a pea-size amount of 302 Remedy. If light moisturization is required, use 302 Recovery Plus. For normal to dry skin, choose between 302 Recovery Plus: Intensive or 302 Day/Night (lotions), or 302 Moisturizing Drops (oil). I also like to add little pure vitamin E oil around my eyes as a finishing touch.

Professional Treatments:

It is a good selfcare practice to get a facial every 6-8 weeks. This includes extractions, if necessary, facial massage, and possibly a stronger ant-aging procedure such as cosmetic ultrasound.

The Youthing Ritual

In TCM, age 35 is when women should begin actively rejuvenating. This includes beginning a more proactive ant-aging skincare regimen and having regular anti-aging treatments. Women who are beginning to see changes in their skin, at any age, should follow this ritual. Women who are experiencing wrinkles, fine lines, loss of skin tone, and thinning skin can use this ritual to begin reversing the damage.

Morning:

Cleansing

The skin should be cleansed 1-2 times a day. The morning requires only a quick, light cleanse or a rinse with cool water. 302 Face & Body Bar is a good choice.

Hydration

Skin typically gets drier as we age. Proper hydration makes our skin look younger. Apply a little 302 Eye Firming Serum around the eyes. Choose between 302 Recovery Plus: Intensive or 302 Day/Night (lotions), or 302 Moisturizing Drops (oil) as your moisturizer.

Sun Protection

Mist with 302 Calming Mist, then apply a thin layer of 302 SPF-30: Tinted.

Evening:

Cleansing

The evening requires more thorough cleansing to remove dirt, pollutants, and make-up. You will wash twice. Apply a dime-size amount of 302 Cleanser (lotion) with dry fingers on dry skin. Massage into the skin to bind to impurities. Then wet your fingers and apply another dime-size amount, massaging into your skin. Rinse thoroughly until there is no more slick.

If you wear make-up, use 302 Normal/ Dry Cleanser in the same manner as 302 Cleanser.

Actives

Begin with 302 C-Boost (1 pump) 3 times per week. Introduce 302 Drops or Serum (1 pump) on alternating nights, working up to 3 times per week. Finally, add 302 A-Boost (1 pump) once per week.

Dull skin; may have thin skin with fine lines. Begin with 302 Plus Drops or Serum (1 pump) every other night. Work up to 5 nights per week. Then add 302 Clarity (a pea-size amount) once a week. Take 1 night per week off from any actives.

Severe sun damage or deep wrinkles. Use 302 Clarity (pea-size amount) 1-2 times a week. Use 302 Drops or Serum on other nights.

Hydration

If light moisturization is required, use

302 Recovery Plus. For normal to dry skin, choose between 302 Recovery Plus: Intensive or 302 Day/Night (lotions), or 302 Moisturizing Drops (oil). I also like to add little pure vitamin E oil around my eyes as a finishing touch.

Professional Treatments:

Professional anti-aging treatments are important to keep the skin young. Frequency depends on the condition of the skin. Cosmetic acupuncture, ultrasound, microcurrent, galvanic, nanocurrent, facial endermologie, and any combination thereof, provide non-irritating, non-damaging stimulation to the skin. Occasional microdermabrasion, peels, or other exfoliation treatments can also be effective to increase cell turnover, as long as skin is not too thin or fragile.

The Skin Brightening Ritual

Hyperpigmentation (dark spots, cholasma) takes time to resolve. This is an intense ritual that should be used for a 3 month duration during times with low sun exposure, typically fall and winter months.

Morning:

Cleansing

The skin should be cleansed 1-2 times a day. The morning requires only a quick, light cleanse or a rinse with cool water. 302 Face & Body Bar is a good choice.

Actives/Hydration

Use 302 Drops or Serum (1 pump) 3 times per week. Alternate with 302 Moisturizing Drops.

Sun Protection

Mist with 302 Calming Mist, then apply a thin layer of 302 SPF-30: Tinted, or 302 SPF-50: Tinted. This will also provide some coverage to even out skin tone.

Evening:

Cleansing

The evening requires more thorough cleansing to remove dirt, pollutants, and make-up. You will wash twice. Apply a dime-size amount of 302 Cleanser (lotion) with dry fingers on dry skin. Massage into the skin to bind to impurities. Then wet your fingers and apply another dime-size amount, massaging into your skin. Rinse thoroughly until there is no more slick.

If your skin is oily, add lather from 302 Face & Body Bar prior to rinsing.

If you make-up, use 302 Normal/Dry Cleanser in the same manner as 302 Cleanser.

Actives

Apply 302 Clarity (pea-size amount) 1-2 times per week. Apply 302 Lightening Drops 3 times per week on alternating nights.

Hydration

Hydration that does not cause dependency or clog pores is an important part of skincare, especially in drier climates. If your skin is normal to oily apply a pea-size amount of 302 Remedy. If light moisturization is required, use 302 Recovery Plus. For normal to dry skin, choose between 302 Recovery Plus: Intensive or 302 Day/Night (lotions), or 302 Moisturizing Drops (oil). I also like to add little pure vitamin E oil around my eyes as a finishing touch.

Professional Treatments:

A series of 6-8 weekly ultrasound or light therapy treatments is very effective to disperse dark spots. Microdermabrasion or peels every 4 weeks or so will help speed cell turnover.

The Clear Skin Ritual

This ritual for acneic conditions including whiteheads, blackheads, pustules, and cystic or nodular acne.

Cleansing

The skin should be cleansed 1-2 times a day. The morning requires only a quick, light cleanse or a rinse with cool water. 302 Face & Body Bar or Sensitive Cleanser Rx are good choices.

Antibacterial & Anti-inflammatory

Apply a thin layer of 302 Revive Rx to all areas with breakouts, being carfeul to avoid the eyes. (This is a great product to wean yourself off benzoyl peroxide). Then apply a pea-size amount of 302 Remedy Rx. The combination of these two products will take down redness, inhibit surface bacteria, and promote wound healing. If you are trying to wean yourself off acids, you can use 302 Enzyme Mist to exfoliate 1-7 times a week.

Oily or teenage skin will typically not require additional moisturization. In cases of adult acne or dry skin, you can apply a moisturizer at this point. If light moisturization is required, use 302 Recovery Plus. For stronger hydration, choose between 302 Recovery Plus: Intensive (lotion), or 302 Moisturizing Drops (oil).

Sun Protection

Many acne suffers rely on excessive make-up to conceal their condition, which causes irritation and blocked pores, compounding the problem. In order to improve your skin more quickly, use instead a pure mineral make-up powder (most of these also provide an SPF of 20 or higher). This can be temporarily uncomfortable, but will speed healing of the condition. 302 Recovery Minerals (SPF-30) is an excellent choice, and there great mineral make-up companies, just be sure to read the ingredients.

If you desire a more dewy finish, apply 1 pump of 302 Moisturizing Drops, mist with Calming Mist, then apply a thin layer of 302 SPF-30: Tinted.

During Sports or Exercise:

If you sweat during the day, you increase the likelihood of breakouts. You can apply a thin layer of 302 Revive Rx before or right after your workout.

Evening:

Pre-Wash

1-4 times per week: apply 302 Sensitive Drops Rx (1 pump) as a mask on acneic areas for 10 minutes. Proceed to cleansing. (If 302 Clarity or 302 A-Boost causes dryness or irritation they can also be used as a mask then washed off on alternating evenings, 1-3 times per week).

Cleansing

The evening requires more thorough cleansing to remove dirt, bacteria, and make-up. You will wash twice. Apply a dime-size amount of 302 Acne Cleanser Rx or 302 Sensitive Cleanser Rx with dry fingers on dry skin. Massage into the skin to bind to impurities. Then wet your fingers and apply another dime-size amount, massaging into your skin. Rinse thoroughly until there is no more slick. If your skin is oily, add lather from 302 Face & Body Bar prior to rinsing.

If you wear make-up or have drier skin, use 302 Normal/Dry Cleanser in the same manner as the above cleansers.

Actives

Vitamin A is highly effective to treat acneic conditions.

Thick, oily skin with pustules, blackheads, and/or whiteheads. Use 302 Clarity (pea-size amount) 1-3 times per week, on alternating nights with 302 Sensitive Drops Rx mask. If your skin becomes dry or irritated, apply it as a mask before washing your face. Leave it on for 10 minutes and wash off. If you are on a stronger retinoid, such as Trentinoin (generic name), use it once per week.

Rash-like acne. Mist with 302 Calming Mist. Then apply a pea-size amount of 302 Remedy Rx.

Cystic acne. Use 302 Clarity (pea-size amount) 1-3 times per week, on alternating nights with 302 Sensitive Drops Rx mask.

Hormonal breakouts. Instead of using 302 Sensitive Drops Rx as a mask, use 302 Drops or 302 Serum. Apply 1 pump to the entire face, neck, and décolleté, and any areas with breakouts, 4-5 times per week. Use 302 A-Boost 1-2 times per week. Spot treat breakouts nightly.

Hydration

Hydration that does not cause dependency or clog pores is an important part of skincare, especially in drier climates. If your skin is normal to oily, apply a pea-size amount of 302 Remedy Rx. If light moisturization is required, use 302 Recovery Plus. For normal to dry skin, choose between 302 Recovery Plus: Intensive (lotion), or 302 Moisturizing Drops (oil). I also like to add little pure vitamin E oil around my eyes as a finishing touch.

Professional Treatments:

Cupping and acupuncture are effective in treating all types of acne when combined with other targeted treatments. A series of colonics may also be effective if there is chronic constipation.

Thick, oily skin with pustules, blackheads, and/or whiteheads. Regular extractions are critical, spaced every 1-2 weeks depending on the severity of the case. Exfoliation treatments, such as microdermabrasion or salicylic acid peels, can be spaced as close as 10 days apart if your skin tolerates this well. Lasers offer an expensive, but effective alternative.

Rash-like acne. The skin is often too senstive for exfoliation treatments. Lymphatic drainage massage on the face or facial endermologie can be helpful. A compress of colloidal silver can be applied twice daily for 10 minutes at a time to alleviate symptoms.

Cystic acne. Severe cystic or nudular acne can cause pitting scars, which are difficult to improve after the fact. In cases in which scarring is probable, I support using Accutane (under a physician's care), to hault the progression.[2] This buys time in which to fix diet, lifestyle, and other areas that may be out of balance. I also recommend using milk thistle tincture during and after Accutane treatment to protect and cleanse

---

2. I am not a physician, so I am only expressing my opinion as someone who has experienced and observed these treatments. I have found internal antibiotic use to be ineffectual longterm, and potentially cause lonterm digestive and immune issues. Though Accutane is a harsh drug, I think it can be worth it when permanent scarring is the alternative.

the liver. Liver toxicity is the major source for side effects from Accutane.

Hormonal breakouts. Acupuncture and Chinese herbs can be used to help balance your cycles. A sluggish lymphatic system is the culprit of many pre-period symptoms, thus facial endermologie or lymphatic drainage massage on the face is effective in many cases when timed a week prior to menstruation.

Pitting acne scars. These scars are difficult to resolve, but with patience and persistence, can be greatly improved. Take Avogen™ capsules daily for 9 months-1 year. A topical product containing the 302 molecule should be used regularly as well. Microneedling (with 302 topicals) can be performed every 6 weeks or so, depending on the depth, for 9 months-1 year. Weekly ultrasound and/or facial endermologie treatments help to soften scar tissue and speed results.

Dark spots that linger post-breakouts. See Skin Brightening Ritual above.

The Calming Ritual

This ritual addresses inflamed, sensitive skin such

as rosacea. The most important thing is to avoid irritants such as acids, detergents, and fragrances, even essential oils.

Cleansing

> The skin should be cleansed 1-2 times a day. The morning requires only a quick, light cleanse with 302 Sensitive Cleanser Rx[3] or a rinse with cool water.

Hydration

> Mist with 302 Calming Mist Rx. Apply a pea-size amount of 302 Remedy Rx to your skin. If your skin requires more moisture, apply 1 pump of 302 Moisturizing Drops Rx.

Sun Protection

> When skin is red and inflamed it is more sensitive to sun damage. Use Recovery Minerals: (SPF-30) as both sunscreen and light make-up.

Evening:

Cleansing

> The evening requires more thorough cleansing to remove dirt, irritants, and make-up. You will wash twice. Apply a dime-size amount of 302 Acne Cleanser Rx

3. Rx means that it does not contain essential oils or other fragrances.

with dry fingers on dry skin. Massage into the skin to bind to impurities. Then wet your fingers and apply another dime-size amount, massaging into your skin. Rinse thoroughly until there is no more slick.

If your skin is oily, add lather from 302 Face & Body Bar Rx prior to rinsing.

Actives

Mist with 302 Calming Mist Rx. Apply 1 pump of 302 Sensitive Drops Rx to your skin beginning every other night, working up to every night. Apply a pea-size amount of 302 Remedy Rx to your skin.

Hydration

If your skin requires more moisture, apply 1 pump of 302 Moisturizing Drops Rx.

Professional Treatments:

Avoid exfoliating treatments. LED light therapy and/or facial endermologie, spaced weekly, can help bring down redness rapidly.

Low Maintenance Rituals

Preventive
- 302 Face & Body Bar twice daily to cleanse
- 302 Recovery Minerals (SPF-30) in the morning after cleansing
- 302 Drops in the evening after cleansing

Acne:
- 302 Face & Body Bar twice daily to cleanse
- 302 Revive Rx in the morning after cleansing and after workouts
- 302 Clarity 1-3 x a week in the evening after cleansing

Anti-aging:
- 302 Cleanser twice daily to cleanse
- 302 Recovery Minerals (SPF-30) in the morning after cleansing
- 302 Plus Drops or Serum 6x a week in the evening after cleansing
- 302 Intensive Recovery: Plus as needed for hydration

Rosacea:
- 302 Sensitive Cleanser Rx twice daily to cleanse
- 302 Recovery Minerals (SPF-30) in the morning after cleansing
- 302 Calming Mist Rx with 302 Remedy Rx twice daily after cleansing

- 302 Moisturizing Drops Rx as needed for hydration

Body Ritual

- exfoliate daily with a body brush or loofah
- use a little 302 Body Treatment: Intensive when you get out of the shower
- oil your body 1-3 times per week with 302 Body Massage Oil as a deep hydration treatment

Professional Treatments:

Body endermologie and ultrasound treatments help keep the lymphatic system healthy and the skin firm.

This is end of a quick guide to natural skincare. I hope this helps you on your journey to optimizing your skin with natural products.

Resources

Skincare

302 Professional Skincare:
> www.302skincare.com
> info@302skincare.com
> tel. (800) 295-7839
> PO Box 2867, Hayden, ID 83835 USA

Chinese Herbs

Chinese herbs can be purchased from licensed acupuncturists.

Wing Hop Fung:
> www.WingHopFung.com (Chinese herbs, teas, and dried foods)

Dragon Herbs:
> www.DragonHerbs.com (Chinese herbs)

Chinese Ingredients

99 Ranch Market:
> www.99Ranch.com. Stores in California, Nevada, Washington, and Texas.

Mitsuwa Market (Japanese):
> www.mitsuwa.com/english/index.html.
> Stores in California, New Jersey and
> Chicago.

Nijiya Market (Japanese):
> www.nijiya.com. Stores in California, New
> York, and Hawaii.

Credits

Cover
Cover Design by Lia Andrews

Interior
Content Editing by Judith Andrews
Layout Design by PXP Design

Index

A

acne , ix, 11, 13, 16, 17, 25, 29, 30, 36, 40, 42, 43, 48, 51, 52, 53, 73, 58, 59, 74, 76, 77, 78, 79, 80
acupuncture 12, 70, 77
adrenals 21
alpha hydroxy acids (AHAs) 58
ammonia polymer 52
anti-aging 14, 82
ascorbic acid 49
avocado oil 55
Avocatin 302 39, 40, 41, 45, 46
Avogen™ 37, 39, 40, 41, 45, 47, 79

B

bacteria 34, 51, 73, 75
bee pollen 34
benzoyl peroxide 11, 15, 52, 73
beta hydroxy acid 58
biotin 42
blackheads 73, 76, 77
black sesame seeds 32
blood deficiency 35
bromelain 58
BV-OSC 49

C

carbamide phosphate 53
chemical sunscreens 59
cholasma 43, 70
cholasma 15, 37
cocoa butter 55
coconut oil 55
collagen 14, 34, 41
colloidal silver 53
confidence 25
cosmetic acupuncture 70
cupping 77
cystic or nodular acne 73

D

dark spots 15, 37, 40, 49, 58, 70, 73
dermis 16, 37, 46, 50
dry Skin 35

E

ECGC in green tea 52
essential oils 80
exercise 22, 24, 75, 76
extractions 67, 77

F

facial endermologie 70, 78, 79, 81

G

galvanic 70
go ji berries 31

H

honey 33
hormonal breakouts 76, 79
hyperpigmentation 13, 15, 37, 40, 43, 48, 49, 58

I

inflammation 13, 17, 18, 36, 42, 51, 53, 58

J

jing 13
jojoba oil 54
jujube dates 32

K

kelp (kombu seaweed) 42
keratin 41

L

light therapy 73, 81
longan berries 31
LOXL 14, 15, 16, 17

lysyl oxidase 14, 17

M

make-up 64
microcirculation 13, 24
microcurrent 70
microdermabrasion 58, 70, 78
milk thistle tincture 43
mulberries 32
multivitamin 41
mushrooms 33

N

nanocurrent 70
niacinamide 50

O

omega 3 fatty acids 42

P

papain 58
pearl powder 43
peels 70, 73, 78
pitting acne scars 79
probiotics 36
Products
   302 A-Boost 49, 66, 69, 75, 77
   302 Acne Cleanser Rx 53,

75, 80
302 Body Massage Oil 83
302 Body Treatment:
   Intensive 48, 83
302 Calming Mist 52, 66,
   68, 71, 76, 80, 81
302 C-Boost 50, 66, 69
302 Clarity 49, 69, 72, 75,
   76, 82
302 Day/Night 54, 55, 56,
   65, 67, 68, 70, 72
302 Drops or Serum 47,
   69, 71
302 Enzyme Mist 58, 74
302 Eye Firming Serum
   51, 65, 68
302 Face & Body Bar 48,
   65, 66, 68, 71, 72,
   73, 76, 81, 82
302 Lightening Drops
   50, 72
302 Moisturizing Drops
   54, 55, 65, 67, 68,
   69, 71, 72, 74, 77,
   80, 81, 83
302 Normal/Dry Cleanser
   64, 66, 69, 72, 76
302 Plus Drops or Serum
   47, 50, 69, 82
302 Recovery Minerals
   (SPF-30) 57, 74,
   75, 82
302 Recovery Plus 54, 55,
   56, 65, 67, 68, 70,
   72, 74, 77
302 Recovery Plus:
   Intensive 54, 55, 56,
   65, 67, 68, 70, 72,
   74, 77
302 Remedy Rx 52, 73,

76, 77, 80, 81, 82
302 Revive Rx 53, 59, 73,
   75, 82
302 Sensitive Cleanser Rx
   75, 80, 82
302 Sensitive Drops 47,
   75, 76, 81
302 SPF-15, 30, & 50 57
302 Treatment Mask 53
Avogen™ Avocado Topical
   Mist 47
propolis 34
pustules 73, 76, 77

Q

qi 13

R

relaxation 22
retinaldehyde 48
retinoic acid 48
retinol 48
retinyl acetate 48
retinyl palmitate 48, 49
rosacea 13, 25, 29, 51, 52,
   53, 80
royal jelly 34

S

salicylic acid
   (carboxyphenol) 58
selenium 42
sensitive skin 79

shea butter 56
sleep 21
sugar 30, 36
sulfates 60
sulfur 53

Y

yang 23, 24
yin 23, 25, 35
youthfulness 25

T

tetrahexydecylascorbate
(THDCA) 49
titanium dioxide 57
toxicity 13, 35, 36, 57, 79
Traditional Chinese
Medicine (TCM) 13

Z

zinc 42, 51, 57
zinc oxide 51, 57

U

ultrasound 67, 70, 79, 80,
83

V

Vitamin B3 50
Vitamin C 42, 49, 50, 66
Vitamin E 42

W

water 29, 30, 35, 36, 42, 49,
65, 68, 71, 73, 80
whiteheads 73, 76, 77
wrinkles 35

About the Author

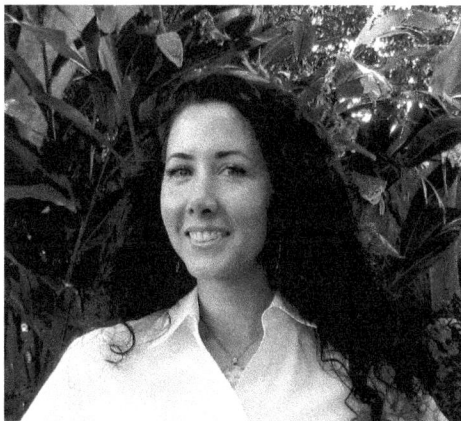

Dr. Lia G. Andrews, DAOM, L.Ac. was born in Norwalk, Connecticut. She attended Bryn Mawr College and the College of William & Mary, where she received her BA in International Studies. She received her Masters in Acupuncture and Traditional Chinese Medicine (MATCM) from Yo San University. Dr. Andrews received her Doctorate of Acupuncture and Oriental Medicine (DAOM) from Pacific College of Oriental Medicine. She is licensed nationally and in the state of California. Also in print is her doctoral capstone on traditional postpartum care: "Partial Translation of 'Postpartum Recovery Program; a Manual of Rules and Recipes for the Postpartum Woman.'" (DAOM capstone, Pacific College of Oriental Medicine, 2013).

Dr. Andrews has traveled to Brazil, Thailand, and China in her study for natural healing. She practices in the clinic she founded with her mother, Dr. Judith Andrews, Cinnabar Acupuncture Clinic & Spa in San Diego, California.

Also Available from Dr. Andrews

Health Awakening Series

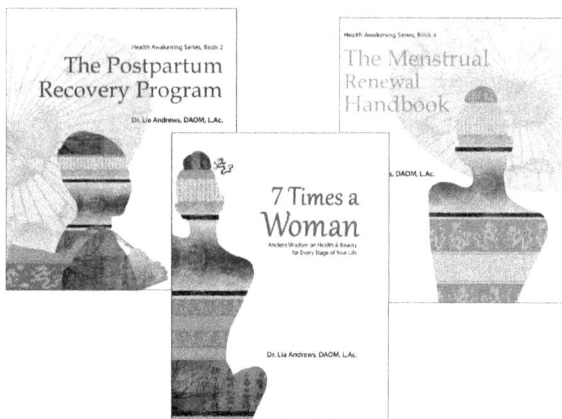

Book 1 - 7 Times a Woman
Book 2 - The Postpartum Recovery Program™

UPCOMING:
Book 3 - The Menstrual Renewal Handbook
Book 4 - Secrets of the Daoist Courtesan
Book 5 - Return to Spring (Menopause)
Book 6 - Detoxification
Book 7 - Empowerment

www.ingramcontent.com/pod-product-compliance
Lightning Source LLC
Chambersburg PA
CBHW050549280326
41933CB00011B/1781